Kidney Disease Dog Treats

And

Cookbook

A Comprehensive Guide with 65 Homemade Recipes to Reverse Kidney Problems in Dogs and Heal Any Underlying Causes

Peter Michtor

Table of Contents

Introduction

In the heartwarming world of our four legged companions, the bond between humans and dogs transcends the ordinary, reaching deep into the world of care, love, and shared moments. Yet, as our loyal friends age, they may encounter health challenges that require our thoughtful attention. One such challenge that often surfaces is kidney disease, a condition that can impact a dog's overall wellbeing.

Welcome to Kidney Disease Dog Treats and Cookbook, a comprehensive guide crafted with love and expertise to help you navigate the intricate landscape of caring for dogs with kidney disease. Within these pages, we embark on a culinary adventure tailored to support your furry friend's health, ensuring that every treat and meal is not just a delight to their taste buds but also a source of nourishment tailored to their specific needs.

As we delve into the pages of this cookbook, you'll discover a treasure trove of recipes designed with simplicity and effectiveness in mind. From scrumptious treats that make training sessions a joy to nutritious meals that prioritize kidney health, each recipe is a testament to the commitment we share with our canine companions.

But Kidney Disease Dog Treats and Cookbook is more than just a collection of recipes; it's a compassionate companion on your journey as a pet parent. We'll explore the fundamentals of kidney disease, demystifying the complexities and providing practical insights into managing your dog's condition. From understanding dietary restrictions to embracing lifestyle changes, this book empowers you to become in Shape and a nurturing advocate for your pet.

Throughout these pages, you'll find not only the science behind kidney friendly nutrition but also the heartwarming stories of other pet parents who have walked a similar path. Their experiences, coupled with expert advice, create a community of support that reassures you that you're not alone in this journey.

Kidney Disease Dog Treats and Cookbook is an invitation to transform meal times into moments of healing; strengthening the connection you share with your dog. Together, let's embark on this culinary and caregiving adventure, ensuring that every wag of the tail is a testament to the love, care, and dedication you pour into your furry friend's life.

Causes of Kidney Disease in Dogs

1. Aging:

Just like people, dogs' organs, particularly the kidneys, may not operate as well as they should as they age. Over time, kidney problems may result from this normal aging process.

2. Genetics:

Because of their genetic composition, certain dog breeds are more likely to experience kidney issues. It's similar to inherited features from parents, only in this instance, the kidneys are involved.

3. Infections:

Pathogenic bacteria can infiltrate a dog's body, leading to infections that occasionally affect the kidneys. It resembles an intruding party guest causing mayhem.

4. Toxic Substances:

Due to their natural curiosity, dogs occasionally eat inappropriate foods. Their kidneys may be harmed by certain chemicals, foods, or plant toxins. It's similar to consuming spicy food but much more serious.

5. Unhealthy Diet:

Dogs require a balanced diet, just like people do. Consuming unhealthy food on a regular basis may cause further strain on their already taxed kidneys.

6. Dehydration:

Can you imagine going days without drinking any water? That's not enjoyable, is it? It's true that dehydration can cause kidney problems in dogs. Staying hydrated is like having a superpower that keeps your kidneys healthy.

7. Medication:

There are occasions when an intended treatment has unintended consequences. Some medications may not work well with a dog's kidneys, leading to problems. It's similar to taking medication that relieves certain symptoms but not others.

8. High Blood Pressure:

High blood pressure in dogs can damage the kidneys, just like it can in people. It's hard on them, just like when you ask a friend to lift a big weight for an extended period of time.

Don't forget to consult your veterinarian if you observe any behavioral changes in your dog, such as increased thirst, frequent urination, or lethargy

Symptoms

Dog kidney disease can present itself in several ways. The following are some typical symptoms to watch out for:

Digestive System Symptoms:

1. Vomiting, with or without blood
2. Diarrhea
3. Reduced appetite
4. Bad breath
5. Mouth ulcers
6. Dark, tarry stool
7. Bleeding gums

Urinary Tract Symptoms:

1. An increase or decrease in the amount of water consumed
2. Increased or decreased urination

Nervous System Symptoms:

1. Change in behavior due to the blood's buildup of waste materials that affect the nervous system
2. Increased thirst and urination are the first indications of Kidney Disease in dogs. Usually, additional symptoms don't show up until roughly two thirds of the kidney tissue has been lost.

It is vital to visit a veterinarian if you detect any changes in your dog's behavior or physical condition, as these symptoms can also be linked to other health conditions. Your dog's life may be extended by receiving early detection and treatment of kidney disease.

Preventions

Although kidney disease in dogs cannot always be prevented, there are a few things you may do to lower the risk:

Keep Up a Nutritional Diet:

Give your dog a well-balanced food that includes fresh water and lean protein.

Prevent Poisons and Toxins:

Keep chemicals and toxins away from your dog that can damage their kidneys. This includes specific flora, foods (such as avocados and grapes), and products (like antifreeze). Additionally, keep in mind that some over-the-counter medications may be detrimental to your dog's kidneys.

Frequent Vet checks:

Frequent veterinary checks will help identify any potential problems early on. Diagnosing kidney problems, such as kidney obstruction or kidney stones, can be done with CBC blood tests, urine analysis, and sometimes even X-rays.

Drink plenty of water for your dog:

Especially in the summer when the blood supply to the kidneys may be reduced by dehydration1.

Make Your House Dog-Proof:

Store all toxins and poisons out of sight and away from places where your dog is allowed to run wild.

Keep in mind that there is no guarantee that your dog won't get kidney disease, these are only preventive measures.

Why Diets are Essential?

Consider the kidneys in your dog as super heroes that toil away in the background to maintain equilibrium. Now, a specific diet becomes the superhero sidekick, helping those kidneys do their vital job when they're not feeling well. Here's why diets are crucial for helping dogs with kidney disease healing:

1. Reducing Workload:

The kidneys remove surplus material and waste from the blood. A kidney-friendly diet reduces this burden, allowing the less-than-happy kidneys to function without feeling overburdened. It resembles treating them to a spa day as opposed to a strenuous lifting session.

2. Balancing Nutrients:

Consider nutrients as the energy source for your kidneys, the superpowers. With the correct diet, your dog may obtain all the proteins, vitamins, and minerals they need without overindulging in those that could strain their kidneys. It resembles a personalized energy drink, only for canines!

3. Managing Fluids:

Excessive or insufficient fluid intake might provide a challenge for kidneys experiencing distress. By controlling the amount of water your dog consumes, you can prevent dehydration and buildup of extra fluid. It's similar to having a carefully controlled irrigation system for the garden of superhuman kidneys.

4. Blood Pressure Control:

Blood pressure and kidneys are closely related. A diet that is good for the kidneys lowers blood pressure and spares these important organs from further strain. It's similar to having a bodyguard who maintains order in the area of the superhero kidneys.

5. Reducing Toxins:

Some foods may include toxins that exacerbate the kidneys' already difficult work. A kidney-friendly diet makes sure the good stuff is the main focus by carefully choosing items to reduce the amount of these dangerous substances. It's similar to building a secure sanctuary free of ominous lurking villains where superheroes can work.

A specific diet is essentially similar to a custom-fit superhero suit; it offers the proper protection and support, enabling the kidneys to repair and carry out their vital role in maintaining your dog's health. In collaboration with your veterinarian, the appropriate food plays a crucial role in the recuperation process, ensuring that those superhuman kidneys receive the necessary care!

Essential Nutrients

Let's take a closer look at the particular nutrients required for a diet that is kidney-friendly for dogs suffering from kidney disease:

1. Protein:

It is essential to have high-quality, readily digested protein sources. Lean meats like turkey and chicken can be among them. While protein limitation is frequently advised, the importance of quality outweighs quantity. Having enough protein is crucial for preserving both general health and muscle mass.

2. Phosphorus:

Controlling phosphorus intake is essential. Excess phosphorus is difficult for impaired kidneys to filter out, which can cause mineral imbalances and additional kidney stress. Seek for dog diets with reduced phosphorus levels, and if your veterinarian suggests it, take into account phosphorus binders.

3. Sodium (Salt):

Maintaining fluid balance and blood pressure require sodium regulation. The kidneys may be strained as a result of elevated blood pressure and fluid retention brought on by an excess of salt. Generally, a low-sodium diet is advised.

4. Omega3 Fatty Acids:

Often included in fish oil, omega3 fatty acids have anti-inflammatory properties and promote kidney health in general. These may be particularly helpful in reducing the inflammation brought on by kidney disease. To guarantee the proper dosage, you should speak with your veterinarian about supplements.

5. Potassium:

Proper potassium levels are necessary for healthy neuron and muscle function. The key is to strike a balance because some diets that are good for kidneys may have lower potassium content. Both too much and too little can be harmful. Bananas and sweet potatoes are examples of foods that are good sources.

Water:

It's important to stay hydrated. Dogs with kidney disease might consume extra water since it's important to stay hydrated to promote kidney function. Make sure your dog always has access to clean water. Your veterinarian can offer advice on particular hydration objectives.

7. Vitamins:

Make sure your dog is getting the vitamins it needs. Vitamins C and B are very crucial. These should be provided by a balanced diet, but if not, your veterinarian may suggest supplements.

8. Calories:

Keeping an eye on your dog's calorie intake is important, particularly if they are not eating as much. It's critical to maintain a healthy weight for general wellbeing and energy levels.

9. Digestible Carbohydrates:

These carbs might serve as a fantastic source of energy. A diet that is kidney-friendly can contain foods that are easy on the digestive system, such as rice and oats.

10. Antioxidants:

Antioxidants help to fight inflammation and oxidative stress. Antioxidants can be found in fruits and vegetables, but be aware of their phosphorus concentration. Carrots and blueberries are two examples of lower-phosphorus foods.

Keep in mind that every dog is different, and your veterinarian can provide the best advice on creating a diet that takes your dog's particular health condition, kidney disease stage, and any other factors into account. Your cherished dog companion's continued health and wellness are ensured by routine examinations and open contact with your veterinarian.

Kidney Disease Dog Treats

These are a list of 15 simple kidney-friendly dog treats you may make for your pet. These sweets are made with the kidneys in mind, but they still taste good.

1. Chicken Bites and Sweet Potato:

Ingredients:

Skinny, boneless chicken breasts

Mashed and cooked sweet potatoes

Instructions:

1. Fully cook and shred the chicken.

2. Mix the mashed sweet potatoes with the shreds of chicken.

3. Shape little, bite-sized balls and bake until firm.

2. Blueberry and Oat Cookies:

Ingredients:

Fresh blueberries

Oats

Egg

Instructions:

1. Puree the blueberries using a blender.

2. Mix the oats, beaten egg, and blueberry puree.

3. Spoon onto a baking sheet, then bake for golden.

3. Turkey Delight and Carrot:

Ingredients:

Grated carrots

Ground turkey

Instructions:

1. In a pan, brown the ground turkey.

2. Add grated carrots and stir.

3. Shape into small patties and bake until cooked.

4. Pumpkin Peanut Butter Bites:

Ingredients:

Canned Pumpkin

All-natural peanut butter

Oat flour

Instructions:

1. Mix oat flour, peanut butter, and pumpkin together.

2. Shape into small balls and refrigerate until firm.

5. Quinoa Squares and Salmon:

Ingredients:

Canned salmon (drained)

Cooked Quinoa

Instructions:

1. Mix cooked quinoa with canned salmon.

2. Press into a baking dish, then bake until set.

6. Cheesy Zucchini Biscuits:

Ingredients:

Grated zucchini

Low-fat cottage cheese

Whole Wheat Flour

Instructions:

1. Mix flour, cottage cheese, and grated zucchini.

2. Shape into biscuits and bake until golden.

7. Apple and Chicken Jerky:

Ingredients:

Sliced apples

Sliced chicken breast

Instructions:

1. Arrange the chicken and apple slices on a baking sheet.

2. Bake until jerky-like and dried out.

8. Carrots and Turkey Meatballs:

Ingredients:

Ground Turkey

Grated carrots

Instructions:

1. Mix grated carrots with ground turkey.

2. Shape into meatballs, and then bake until cooked through.

9. Spinach and Cottage Cheese Drops:

Ingredients:

Chopped fresh spinach

Low-fat cottage cheese

Brown rice flour.

Instructions:

1. Blend cottage cheese and spinach together, and then mix in brown rice flour.

2. Drop spoonfuls onto a baking sheet and bake.

10. Cranberry and Rice Treats:

Ingredients:

Cooked rice

Unsweetened dried cranberries

Instructions:

1. Mix dried cranberries into cooked rice.

2. Shape into small treats and refrigerate.

11. Beef and Pumpkin Patties:

Ingredients:

Lean ground beef

Canned Pumpkin

Instructions:

1. Ground beef is browned and mixed with canned pumpkin.

2. Shape into patties and bake until cooked.

12. Pea and Chicken Cookies:

Ingredients:

Frozen mashed peas

Shredded cooked chicken

Instructions:

1. Mash peas and mix with shredded chicken.

2. Shape into cookie shapes, and then bake until firm.

13. Sweet Potato and Turkey Roll-Ups:

Ingredients:

Cooked and mashed sweet potatoes

Sliced turkey

Instructions:

1. Top turkey slices with mashed sweet potatoes.

2. Slice into bite-sized pieces after rolling up.

14. Broccoli and Salmon Bites:

Ingredients:

Broccoli, finely chopped and steam-cooked

Canned Salmon (drained)

Instructions:

1. Mix canned salmon with chopped broccoli.

2. Shape into small balls and bake.

15. Carob and Banana Popsicles:

Ingredients:

Mashed banana

Carob powder

Instructions:

1. Mix carob powder and mashed banana.

2. Freeze in little molds to enjoy a refreshing summer treat.

Don't forget to gradually introduce new treats to your dog and keep an eye out for any negative reactions.

Kidney Disease Dog Diets

These are dog diets that are kidney friendly, along with ingredients and instructions. As each dog is different, always check with your veterinarian before making any major dietary changes. Always remember to introduce new foods gradually to prevent upset stomach.

1. Chicken and Rice Delight:

Ingredients

Carrots

White rice

Boiled chicken.

Instructions:

Cook chicken until cooked through, shred it, then Mix it with finely chopped carrots and cooked rice.

2. Turkey and Sweet Potato Stew:

Ingredients

Sweet potatoes

Green beans

Ground Turkey.

Instructions:

After browning the turkey, add diced sweet potatoes and green beans, simmer until veggies are tender.

3. Fish and Quinoa Medley:

Ingredients:

Quinoa

Peas

Baked white fish, such as cod.

Instructions:

Cook the quinoa and peas, then bake the fish and flake it, and mix with cooked quinoa and peas.

4. Beef and Barley Casserole:

Ingredients:

Barley

Spinach

Lean ground beef.

Instructions:

Cook the barley, add the cooked barley and chopped spinach and stir until the spinach wilts.

5. Chicken and Pumpkin Porridge:

Ingredients:

Brown rice

Cooked chicken

Pumpkin.

Instructions:

Mix cooked brown rice, mashed pumpkin, and shredded chicken.

6. Turkey and Carrot Patties:

Ingredients:

Ground turkey

Grated carrots

Oats.

Instructions:

Mix shredded carrots, oats, and ground turkey. Shape into patties, and then bake.

7. Salmon and Potato Hash:

Ingredients:

Baked salmon

Boiled potatoes

Green peas.

Instructions:

Diced boiled potatoes and green peas should be mixed with flake baked salmon.

8. Vegetable Lentil Stew:

Ingredients:

Sweet potatoes

Zucchini

Lentils.

Instructions:

Add chopped sweet potatoes and zucchini to cooked lentils and simmer until veggies are tender.

9. Chicken and Brown Rice Casserole:

Ingredients:

Brown rice

Broccoli

Chicken thighs.

Instructions:

Bake chicken thighs, shred, and mix cooked brown rice and steamed broccoli.

10. Turkey and Mash Cauliflower:

Ingredients:

Carrots

Cauliflower

Ground turkey.

Instructions:

Brown the turkey, mash the cauliflower, and then stir in the chopped carrots.

11. Tuna and Rice Surprise:

Ingredients:

Green beans

White rice

Canned tuna in water.

Instructions:

Drain tuna and mix with finely chopped green beans and cooked rice.

12. Chicken and Quinoa Bowl:

Ingredients:

Grilled chicken breast

Quinoa

Peas.

Instructions:

Cook the quinoa and peas, then chop and toss with the grilled chicken.

13. Beef and Pumpkin Stew:

Ingredients:

Brown rice

Pumpkin

Lean beef chunks.

Instructions:

Brown beef chunks, add cooked brown rice and diced pumpkin, and simmer until pumpkin is soft.

14. Salmon and Spinach Delight:

Ingredients:

Sweet potatoes

Spinach

Baked salmon.

Instructions:

Flake the baked salmon and mix it with the mashed sweet potatoes and chopped spinach.

15. Turkey and Barley Bake:

Ingredients:

Carrots

Barley

Ground turkey.

Instructions:

Cook the barley, add the diced carrots and brown the turkey; bake until the carrots are soft.

16. Chicken and Green Bean Saute:

Ingredients:

Brown rice

Cooked chicken

Green beans.

Instructions:

Saute cooked brown rice and green beans with cooked chicken.

17. Fish and Carrots Stir-fry:

Ingredients:

Carrots

Quinoa

Baked fish.

Instructions:

Flake baked fish, stir-fry with sliced carrots and cooked quinoa.

18. Beef and Broccoli Bowl:

Ingredients:

Sweet potatoes

Broccoli

Lean beef strips.

Instructions:

Stir-fry beef strips with broccoli, mix in mashed sweet potatoes.

19. Chicken and Zucchini Medley:

Ingredients:

Brown rice

Zucchini

Grilled chicken.

Instructions:

Grill chicken, slice, mix with sautéed zucchini and cooked brown rice.

20. Turkey and Pumpkin Soup:

Ingredients:

Barley

Pumpkin

Ground turkey.

Instructions:

Brown the turkey, then add the cooked barley and diced pumpkin. Simmer with water to make a soup.

Keep an eye on how your dog responds to these diets, and if in doubt, ask your veterinarian for advice on portion quantities and how to adjust for your dog's particular needs.

21. Low-Phosphorus Dog Food:

Ingredients:

Ground beef, long-grain rice, egg, sunflower oil, calcium carbonate, di-calcium phosphate, fish oil, salt, potassium chloride, choline chloride, zinc sulfate, ferrous sulfate, vitamin E supplement, copper sulfate, vitamin B12 supplement, and vitamin A supplement.

Instructions:

Cook rice and ground beef separately. After cooked, Mix all ingredients in a big bowl. Serve at room temperature.

22. Chicken and Pumpkin Stew:

Ingredients:

Fish oil, peas, carrots, pumpkin, and boneless chicken.

Instructions:

Bring the chicken to a boil until it is tender. Steam the carrots, peas, and pumpkin until they are tender. Mix all ingredients and serve.

23. Fish and Sweet Potato Diet:

Ingredients:

Fish oil, sweet potatoes, green beans, and white fish.

Instructions:

Cook the sweet potatoes and fish completely by steaming them. Mix all ingredients and serve.

24. Turkey and Quinoa Meal:

Ingredients:

Fish oil, carrots, peas, and ground turkey.

Instructions:

Cook the quinoa and ground turkey separately. After cooked, Mix all ingredients in a big bowl. Serve at room temperature.

25. Beef and Rice Diet:

Ingredients:

Fish oil, carrots, peas, brown rice, and lean ground beef.

Instructions:

Cook rice and ground beef separately. After cooked, Mix all ingredients in a big bowl. Serve at room temperature.

26. Lamb and Barley Diet:

Fish oil, peas, zucchini, barley, and ground lamb.

Instructions:

Cook the barley and ground lamb separately. After cooked, Mix all ingredients in a big bowl. Serve at room temperature.

27. Chicken and Couscous Meal:

Fish oil, carrots, peas, couscous, and boneless chicken.

Instructions:

Bring the chicken to a boil until it is tender. Follow the directions on the package to prepare the couscous. Mix all ingredients and serve.

28. Salmon and Rice Diet:

Fish oil, brown rice, green beans, and salmon.

Instructions:

Steam the rice and fish separately until they are thoroughly cooked. Mix all ingredients and serve.

29. Turkey and Sweet Potato Meal:

Fish oil, sweet potatoes, peas, and carrots.

Instructions:

Cook sweet potatoes and ground turkey in separate pans. After cooked, Mix all ingredients in a big bowl. Serve at room temperature.

30. Beef and Quinoa Diet:

Fish oil, carrots, peas, quinoa, and lean ground beef.

Instructions:

Cook the quinoa and ground beef separately. After cooked, Mix all ingredients in a big bowl. Serve at room temperature.

31. Chicken and Barley Diet:

Fish oil, barley, carrots, peas, and boneless chicken.

Instructions:

Bring the chicken to a boil until it is tender. Follow the package's instructions to cook the barley. Mix all ingredients and serve.

32. Fish and Quinoa Meal:

White fish, peas, quinoa, zucchini, and fish oil.

Instructions:

Cook the quinoa and fish separately in the steamer until they are done. Mix all ingredients and serve.

33. Turkey and Rice Diet:

Fish oil, brown rice, green beans, and ground turkey.

Instructions:

Cook the rice and the ground turkey separately. After cooked, Mix all ingredients in a big bowl. Serve at room temperature.

34. Beef and Couscous Meal:

Fish oil, carrots, peas, and lean ground beef.

Instructions:

Cook the couscous and ground beef in separate pans. After cooked, Mix all ingredients in a big bowl. Serve at room temperature.

35. Lamb and Sweet Potato Diet:

Fish oil, sweet potatoes, peas, carrots, and ground lamb.

Instructions:

Cook sweet potatoes and ground lamb in separate pans. After cooked, Mix all ingredients in a big bowl. Serve at room temperature.

36. Chicken and Sweet Potato Meal:

Fish oil, sweet potatoes, zucchini, peas, and boneless chicken.

Instructions:

Bring the chicken to a boil until it is tender. Follow the directions on the package to cook the sweet potatoes. Mix all ingredients and serve.

37. Fish and Barley Diet:

Fish oil, barley, green beans, and white fish.

Instructions:

Steam the barley and fish separately until they are cooked through. Mix all ingredients and serve.

38. Turkey and Couscous Meal:

Fish oil, carrots, peas, couscous, and ground turkey.

Instructions:

Cook the couscous and ground turkey in separate pans. After cooked, Mix all ingredients in a big bowl. Serve at room temperature.

39. Beef and Sweet Potato Diet:

Fish oil, sweet potatoes, carrots, peas, and lean ground beef.

Instructions:

Cook sweet potatoes and ground meat in separate pans. After cooked, Mix all ingredients in a big bowl. Serve at room temperature.

40. Lamb and Rice Meal:

Fish oil, peas, carrots, brown rice, and ground lamb.

Instructions:

Cook the rice and the ground lamb separately. After cooked, Mix all ingredients in a big bowl. Serve at room temperature.

41. Chicken and Quinoa Diet:

Fish oil, peas, carrots, quinoa, and boneless chicken.

Instructions:

Bring the chicken to a boil until it is tender. Follow the directions on the package to prepare the quinoa. Mix all ingredients and serve.

42. Fish and Couscous Meal:

Green beans, couscous, white fish, and fish oil.

Instructions:

Steam the couscous and fish separately until they are cooked through. Mix all ingredients and serve.

43. Turkey and Barley Diet:

Fish oil, carrots, peas, barley, and ground turkey.

Instructions:

Cook the barley and ground turkey separately. After cooked, Mix all ingredients in a big bowl. Serve at room temperature.

44. Beef and Quinoa Meal:

Fish oil, peas, zucchini, and lean ground beef.

Instructions:

Cook the quinoa and ground beef separately. After cooked, Mix all ingredients in a big bowl. Serve at room temperature.

45. Lamb and Couscous Diet:

Ground lamb, couscous, peas, carrots, and fish oil.

Instructions:

Cook the couscous and ground lamb separately. After cooked, Mix all ingredients in a big bowl. Serve at room temperature.

46. Chicken and Sweet Potato Stew:

Fish oil, peas, carrots, sweet potatoes, and boneless chicken.

Instructions:

Bring the chicken to a boil until it is tender. Let the carrots, peas, and sweet potatoes steam until tender. Mix all ingredients and serve.

47. Fish and Rice Meal:

Fish oil, peas, zucchini, brown rice, and white fish.

Instructions:

Cook the rice and fish separately in the steam oven until they are done. Mix all ingredients and serve.

48. Turkey and Sweet Potato Diet:

Sweet potatoes, peas, carrots, ground turkey, and fish oil.

Instructions:

Cook sweet potatoes and ground turkey in separate pans. After cooked, Mix all ingredients in a big bowl. Serve at room temperature.

49. Beef and Barley Meal:

Fish oil, barley, zucchini, peas, and lean ground beef.

Instructions:

Cook barley and ground beef separately. After cooked, Mix all ingredients in a big bowl. Serve at room temperature.

50. Lamb and Quinoa Diet:

Fish oil, quinoa, carrots, peas, and ground lamb.

Instructions:

Prepare the quinoa and ground lamb separately. After cooked, Mix all ingredients in a big bowl. Serve at room temperature.

How to Care for a Sick Dog

A sick dog needs love, care, and appropriate medical attention in addition to other necessities. This is an exhaustive guide that will assist you in providing for your pet throughout their disease:

1. Consult the Veterinarian:

Early Detection: Be alert for indicators of disease, such as behavioral, eating, or toilet changes. See your veterinarian right away if you detect anything strange.

Frequent Checkups: Plan routine veterinary examinations to keep an eye on your dog's general health and identify any potential problems early.

2. Establish a Cozy Environment:

Calm Environment: Give your sick dog a peaceful, cozy place to recuperate. To reduce stress, make sure it's far from other animals and loud noises.

Bedding: Make use of cozy, machine-washable bedding. To keep everything hygienic, clean and replace it frequently.

3. Hydration:

Fresh Water: Consistently provide your dog with access to clean water. Staying well hydrated is essential for healing.

Hydration Monitoring: Pay attention to how much water your dog consumes. Speak with your veterinarian if there is a noticeable decline.

4. Administration of Medication:

Observe the advice of the veterinarian: Follow your veterinarian's instructions precisely when giving prescribed medication. Follow the suggested dosage and timetable.

Pose inquiries: Ask your veterinarian for clarification if you have any questions regarding the medication.

5. Nutrition:

Special Diet: Adhere strictly to your veterinarian's recommendations if one is given for your sick dog. Nutritional supplements may help in healing.

Monitoring Appetite: Watch how hungry your dog is. See your veterinarian if your pet isn't interested in eating.

6. Keep an eye on your symptoms:

Observation: Observe your dog's symptoms closely. Behavior, respiration, or physiological changes might all be significant markers.

Temperature Monitoring: Learn how to take your dog's temperature and heed your veterinarian's advice on how to treat it if it has a fever.

7. Tidying and Personal Hygiene:

Continual Personal Care: Regular grooming will keep your dog clean and help avoid skin problems. This is particularly crucial if your dog's mobility is compromised while unwell.

Accidents: Clean up spills right away to save your dog from getting sick or uncomfortable.

8. Physical Comfort:

Gentle Exercise: If your veterinarian gives the go-ahead, give your dog mild workouts suitable for its condition. Playtime or quick walks might speed up the healing process.

Pain management: Talk to your veterinarian about pain management techniques if your dog is in discomfort. Medication or physical therapy may be part of this.

9. Support on an Emotional Level:

Kindness: Show a lot of love and kindness. Your comfort and presence can make a big difference in your dog's health.

Patience: Be patient, particularly if your dog's sickness is causing them to become agitated or nervous. They can be calmed by your serene presence.

10. Routine Veterinary Checkups:

Appointments for Follow-Up: Keep the follow-up appointments that your veterinarian has set up. These appointments are crucial for monitoring development and modifying the treatment plan as necessary.

11. Being Ready for Emergencies:

Recognize Emergency Signs: Learn how to recognize emergency or distress indicators. Keep the phone number of your veterinarian and the address of the closest emergency veterinary clinic close at hand.

12. Evaluations of Quality of Life:

Quantity vs. Quality: Check your dog's quality of life on a regular basis. Sometimes the finest thing to do is to give them love and comfort while they're still alive.

13. Look for Assistance:

Veterinary Guidance: If you have any questions or concerns, don't be afraid to call your veterinarian. They are available to assist you in navigating the caregiving process.

Assistance Networks: Make contact with neighborhood or online support organizations for pet owners experiencing comparable circumstances. Support on an emotional level is essential for carers.

Although taking care of a sick dog might be difficult, your commitment and the right treatment can have a big impact on their rehabilitation and general health.

Conclusion

Through the inspiring journey found in Kidney Disease Dog Treats and Cookbook," we've set out on a quest to change mealtimes for our furry friends with kidney difficulties into times of healing, happiness, and steadfast love. This cookbook is more than just a list of recipes; it is evidence of the close relationship we have with our four-legged companions and our extraordinary dedication to their well-being.

We've learned from reading through the pages that cooking kidney-friendly meals and treats is about taking care of our dogs' souls as much as their bodies. Pet owners are empowered to become healers in their own kitchens, offering comfort and care with each delectable bite because to the recipes' simplicity and careful ingredient selection.

We've explored the world of nutrient-rich, kidney-friendly ingredients through these culinary explorations, creating snacks and dishes that have the ideal ratio of taste to utility. Every recipe serves as a chapter in the narrative of perseverance, highlighting the fortitude and versatility of our devoted allies.

More than just a recipe book, "Kidney Disease Dog Treats and Cookbook" is a comprehensive reference that helps readers understand the complexity of kidney disease and provides expert guidance and useful ideas to help them face obstacles head-on. It's a supportive network where other pet parents' shared experiences reaffirm that nobody travels this path alone.

Let this cookbook serve as a source of motivation and empowerment as we come to an end. I hope the recipes in these pages will make your dog happy and content and benefit their health.

Let this book serve as a reminder that our dedication to their well-being is evidence of the ongoing love and friendship that characterizes the wonderful link between people and dogs, as we continue to spend our lives with these amazing creatures.

Cheers to a future full of happy times, treats shared, and the reassurance that we can support our animal friends through every stage of their lives because we have this book at our disposal.

BONUS PAGE

Diets for Dog Owners

One of the best ways to keep yourself and your pet exercise partner happy and fit is to develop a strong and healthy friendship. Here are several bodybuilding recipes with Ingredients and Instructions for dog owners:

1. Protein Packed Power Bites:

Ingredients:

1 cup of ground beef that is lean

½ cup of cooked quinoa

1 beaten egg

Instructions:

1. Fully cook the ground beef.

2. Mix quinoa, beaten egg, and cooked beef.

3. Shape into small, bite-sized balls and bake until cooked through.

2. Sweet Potato and Chicken Muscle Muffins:

Ingredients:

1 cup of shredded cooked chicken

½ cup of mashed sweet potatoes

¼ cup cottage cheese

Instructions:

1. Mix cottage cheese, mashed sweet potato, and shreds of chicken.

2. Fill muffin cups with mixture, and then bake until set.

3. Salmon and Oats Energy Bars:

Ingredients:

1 can of drained canned salmon (in water)

1 cup of rolled oats

¼ cup of grated carrots

Instructions:

1. Grate the carrot and add the oats to the mashed salmon.

2. Transfer the mixture to a baking dish and bake it for a solid result.

59

4. Turkey and Spinach Muscle Wraps:

Ingredients:

1 cup cooked ground turkey

½ cup of finely chopped spinach

Whole wheat tortillas

Instructions:

1. Mix chopped spinach with cooked ground turkey.

2. Transfer the mixture onto whole wheat tortillas, and then roll them up.

5. Beef and Blueberries Protein Smoothie:

Ingredients:

½ cup of chopped cooked beef

½ cup of blueberries

½ cup of plain yogurt

Instructions:

1. Blend the yogurt, blueberries, and cooked beef until smooth.

6. Peanut Butter Banana Power Bites:

Ingredients:

1 cup of mashed bananas

½ cup of natural peanut butter

1 cup of oats

Instructions:

1. Mix peanut butter, oats, and mashed bananas.

2. Shape into small balls and refrigerate until firm.

7. Tuna and Brown Rice Energy Bowl:

Ingredients:

1 can canned (drained) of tuna in water

1 cup of cooked brown rice

¼ cup cooked peas

Instructions:

1. In a bowl, Mix cooked brown rice, peas, and tuna.

8. Chicken and Pumpkin Power Pancakes:

Ingredients:

1 cup of shredded cooked chicken

½ cup of pureed pumpkin

1 egg

Instructions:

1. Mix beaten egg, pureed pumpkin, and shreds of chicken.

2. Use a griddle to cook small pancakes.

9. Sardine and Carrot Crunch Biscuits:

Ingredients:

1 can of mashed canned sardines (in water)

1 cup of grated carrots

1½ cups whole wheat flour

Instructions:

1. Mix whole wheat flour, grated carrots, and mashed sardines.

2. Roll out the dough, cut it into biscuit shapes, and bake them.

10. Turkey and Green Beans Muscle Stir-fry:

Ingredients:

1 cup cooked ground turkey

1 cup of steamed chopped green beans

½ cup of cooked brown rice

Instructions:

1. Stir-fry cooked ground turkey with steamed green beans.

2. Serve over cooked brown rice.

These recipes not only provide delicious treats that you and your dog can enjoy together after an exercise, but they also give your dog the vital nutrients.

Notes

63

Notes

64

Notes

Notes

Notes

67

Notes

Notes

69

Notes

70

www.ingramcontent.com/pod-product-compliance
Lightning Source LLC
Chambersburg PA
CDIIW071056260726
48661CB00006B/2313